Trauma-Informed Care
and
Behavioral Health Services

Achieving Compliance in Long-Term Care

Barbara F. Speedling

© 2019 Barbara F. Speedling
All rights reserved.

TABLE OF CONTENTS

1. Introduction — 4
2. How to Use This Resource Guide — 5
3. Systems to Be Evaluated — 7
4. Steps to Achieving Compliance — 9
5. Trauma-Informed Care — 11
   a. F699 Trauma-Informed Care
   b. F700 Bed Rails
6. Behavioral Health — 15
   a. F740
   b. F741 – Sufficient Staff
   c. F742 – Residents with a History of Trauma
   d. F743 – Residents without a History of Trauma
   e. Resources — 21
      i. Mental Health
      ii. Substance Abuse/Addictions
      iii. Intellectual/Developmental Disability
      iv. Traumatic Brain Injury
   f. F744 - Dementia Care — 22
      i. Staff Education, Training, And Certification
7. F645 Pre-Admission Screening and Resident Review (PASARR) — 25
8. Facility Assessment — 27
9. Evaluating Medication Management/Unnecessary Drugs — 29
10. Attachment A - Regulatory Revisions by Phase — 30
11. References — 33

INTRODUCTION

The Centers for Medicare and Medicaid (CMS) is the Federal agency within the United States Department of Health and Human Services (HHS) that administers the Medicare program and works in partnership with state governments to administer Medicaid. The agency is also responsible for monitoring the quality standards in long-term care facilities through its survey and certification process.

According to the Centers for Disease Control (CDC) 1.6 million people resided in nursing homes in the United States in 2017. Medicare is the primary payer for 52 percent of residents who have been in a nursing home for less than 30 days. A combination of longer life spans and spiraling health care costs has left an estimated 64 percent of the Americans in nursing homes dependent on Medicaid.

In 2016, CMS published the final Rules of Participation for all long-term care facilities. The requirements were revised to reflect the substantial advances that have been made over the past several years in the theory and practice of service delivery and safety. Published in three phases, full compliance with the revisions in all three phases is required by November 28, 2019.
*For a complete list of requirements in each phase, please refer to Attachment A.

The State Operations Manual (SOM), published by CMS, contains guidance to surveyors on evaluating a long-term care facility's compliance with Federal regulations. The survey protocols and interpretive guidelines contained in the manual are intended to clarify the intent of the regulations. Surveyors are required to utilize these tools in evaluating and addressing potential concerns relative to the compliance and quality of care in long-term care facilities.

Organized in several appendices, Appendix PP contains the complete listing of the Federal regulations (F-Tags). This information is found at: https://www.cms.gov/Medicare/Provider-Enrollment-and-Certification/GuidanceforLawsAndRegulations/Nursing-Homes.html

The following five topics are the focus in Phase Three:

1. Freedom from Abuse, Neglect, Mistreatment, and Exploitation;
2. Trauma-Informed Care and Behavioral Health Services;
3. Food and Nutrition Services;
4. Infection Control/Infection Preventionist Program; and
5. Quality Assurance/Performance Improvement

In addition to the guidance provided in SOM Appendix PP, CMS has developed Long-Term Care Survey Pathways[i] as tools for surveyors to use in determining if a facility is providing the necessary care and services required by each individual resident's assessment. Each Pathway evidences the process by which compliance is evaluated:

- Observation and Interview (Across all Shifts)
    - Staff Interviews
    - Resident and Family Interviews
- Policy Review
- Medical Record Review

HOW TO USE THIS RESOURCE GUIDE

This resource guide is designed to assist the interdisciplinary team in understanding the full scope of responsibility under the regulations for Trauma-Informed Care and Behavioral Health Services. Each section offers an overview of the regulatory requirements, highlights on how to interpret the intent of the requirement, and the steps the team will want to focus on to evaluate compliance and identify areas in need of review and potential revision.

The regulations for Trauma-Informed Care (F699-F700) and Behavioral Health Services (F740-F744) introduce new aspects of care and service that few long-term care facilities have had to consider. For example, F699 will require the facility to include an initial screening for Post-Traumatic Stress Disorder (PTSD) for all new admission.

While there is no direct requirement for a screening process or a particular screening tool referenced in F699, the need for this assessment is implied in the language of the regulation. It is later found to be required under F742 Behavioral Health. This highlights the importance of understanding how the regulatory standards are integrated and overlapping in many areas. In this example, without a standardized assessment process, the facility will not be able to show that there is a method for determining if a resident is a trauma survivor at the time of admission.

F699 Trauma-Informed Care

The facility must ensure that residents who are trauma survivors receive culturally competent, trauma-informed care in accordance with professional standards of practice and accounting for residents' experiences and preferences in order to eliminate or mitigate triggers that may cause re-traumatization of the resident.

F742 Behavioral Health
The facility must ensure that a resident who displays or is diagnosed with mental disorder or psychosocial adjustment difficulty, or who has a history of trauma and/or post-traumatic stress disorder, receives appropriate treatment and services to correct the assessed problem or to attain the highest practicable mental and psychosocial well-being;

INTENT §483.40(b) & §483.40(b)(1)

- **Upon admission**, residents assessed or diagnosed with a mental or psychosocial adjustment difficulty or a history of trauma and/or post-traumatic stress disorder (PTSD), receive the appropriate treatment and services to correct the initial assessed problem or to attain the highest practicable mental and psychosocial well-being.

- Residents who were admitted to the nursing home with a mental or psychosocial adjustment difficulty, or who have a history of trauma and/or PTSD, must receive appropriate person-centered and individualized treatment and services to meet their assessed needs.

The challenge to long-term care facilities is to ensure that they are fully prepared to care for a new demographic of residents with complex psychiatric and psychosocial needs. Beyond differentiating dementia from psychiatric illness or addictions, the facility staff must ensure that the staff have a working knowledge of the interventions and services necessary to ensure quality care for a rapidly changing population.

KEY SYSTEMS TO BE EVALUATED

1. **Admission Considerations:**
    a. Capacity Determination (Ref. F600 Abuse – Involuntary Seclusion)
    F600 §483.12 Freedom from Abuse, Neglect, and Exploitation
    - For information related to determining consent, refer to "Assessment of Older Adults with Diminished Capacity: A Handbook for Psychologists" ©
    - American Bar Association Commission on Law and Aging – American Psychological Association, located at:
    http://www.apa.org/pi/aging/programs/assessment/capacity-psychologist-handbook.pdf
    b. Advance Directives (Ref. F578 – Residents' Rights/Advance Directives)
    c. Pre-Admission Screening and Resident Review (PASARR)

2. **Nursing/Medical Considerations:**
    a. Resident/Family Orientation
    b. Admission Assessment/History and Physical
    c. Unnecessary Drugs/Medication Reconciliation
    d. Baseline Care Plan Development and Validation of Resident/Family Receipt
    e. Care Plan Implementation and Oversight
    f. Interdisciplinary Communication and Coordination with Direct Care Staff
        i. Restraints/Side Rails
        ii. Pain Management
        iii. Food and Nutrition
        iv. Dementia Care Standards
        v. Mental Health Services/Community Care Partners
        vi. Substance Abuse/Addiction Assessment and Care Planning
        vii. Care and services for Residents with Intellectual/Developmental Disability
        viii. Care and services for Residents with Traumatic Brain Injury
    g. Palliative/Hospice Services

3. **Social Service Considerations:**
    a. Admission Assessment
    b. Care Plan/Service Coordination
    c. Residents' Rights/Capacity Determination
    d. Advance Directives
    e. Psychotropic Medication/Gradual Dose Reduction
    f. Psychiatric/Psychological Services Coordination
    g. Addiction Services
    h. Resident Education and Support
    i. Family Education and Support
    j. Discharge Planning
    k. Palliative/Hospice Services

4. **Rehabilitation/Recreation Therapy**
    a. Admission Assessment
    b. Care Plan/Service Coordination
    c. Therapeutic Programming
        i. Dementia Classification and Staging
        ii. Mental Health Interventions
        iii. Age-Appropriate Activity
        iv. Education and Self-Help Programming
        v. Community Partners and Volunteer Support
    d. Discharge Planning

STEPS TO ACHIEVING COMPLIANCE

1. Provide all essential staff copies of the Federal regulations for Trauma-Informed Care (F699-F700) and Behavioral Health Services (F740-F744) as required reading;
2. Convene a Quality Assurance/Performance Improvement (QAPI) Committee with all essential staff to review and discuss the Federal regulations;
    a. Create subcommittees responsible for:
        i. Policy review and revision;
        ii. Revision of the Facility Assessment to reflect new and revised care and service protocols (Ref. F838 Facility Assessment);
        iii. Staff education, training, and competency; and
        iv. Development of new services and community partners.
    b. Develop QAPI systems and tools for ongoing monitoring.
3. Utilize the CMS Long-Term Care Survey Pathways to complete full, systemic reviews of all vital care and services relative to compliance in Trauma-Informed Care and Behavioral Health Services:
    a. CMS-20059 Abuse
    b. CMS-20062 Sufficient and Competent Staff
    c. CMS-20065 Activities
    d. CMS-20067 Behavioral-Emotional
    e. CMS-20069 Communication-Sensory
    f. CMS-20076 Pain Management
    g. CMS-20077 Physical Restraints
    h. CMS-20082 Unnecessary Medication
    i. CMS-20090 PASARR (Pre-Admission Screening and Resident Review)
    j. CMS-20127 Accidents
    k. CMS-20130 Neglect
    l. CMS-20131 Resident Assessment
    m. CMS-20133 Dementia Care
4. Provide education and training to all staff on the revisions to facility policy and procedures for compliance with Trauma-Informed Care and Behavioral Health Services;

    a. Revise and/or create ongoing quality monitoring tools to ensure staff remain competent and skilled in the care of the facility's current population; and
    b. Develop education for residents and families on the facility's new and revised policies and procedures.
5. Ensure that all changes to facility care and services are accurately reflected in the Facility Assessment and revised, as needed, when there are shifts in demographics or revisions to the regulatory requirements.

I

F699 TRAUMA-INFORMED CARE

§483.25(m) Trauma-informed care

[§483.25(m) will be implemented beginning November 28, 2019 (Phase 3)]

The facility must ensure that residents who are trauma survivors receive culturally competent, trauma-informed care in accordance with professional standards of practice and accounting for residents' experiences and preferences in order to eliminate or mitigate triggers that may cause re-traumatization of the resident.

F700 §483.25(n) Bed Rails.

[(Effective: 11-28-17, Implementation: 11-28-17)]

The facility must attempt to use appropriate alternatives prior to installing a side or bed rail. If a bed or side rail is used, the facility must ensure correct installation, use, and maintenance of bed rails, including but not limited to the following elements.

§483.25(n)(1) Assess the resident for risk of entrapment from bed rails prior to installation.

§483.25(n)(2) Review the risks and benefits of bed rails with the resident or resident representative and obtain informed consent prior to installation.

§483.25(n)(3) Ensure that the bed's dimensions are appropriate for the resident's size and weight.

§483.25(n)(4) Follow the manufacturers' recommendations and specifications for installing and maintaining bed rails.

What is Trauma-Informed Care?

Trauma-Informed Care understands and considers the pervasive nature of trauma and promotes environments of healing and recovery rather than practices and services that may inadvertently re-traumatize.

INTENT §483.25(n)

The intent of this requirement is to ensure that prior to the installation of bed rails, the facility has attempted to use alternatives; if the alternatives that were attempted were not adequate to meet the resident's needs, the resident is assessed for the use of bed rails, which includes a review of risks including entrapment; and informed consent is obtained from the resident or if applicable, the resident representative. The facility must ensure the bed is appropriate for the resident and that bed rails are properly installed and maintained.

EVALUATE POTENTIAL QUALITY CONCERNS:

- **Accident Hazard** -The resident could attempt to climb over, around, between, or through the rails, or over the foot board;
- **Restraint -** Hinders residents from independently getting out of bed thereby confining them to their beds
- **Behavioral Health** –
    - Creates an undignified self-image and alters the resident's self-esteem;
    - Contributes to feelings of isolation; and
    - Induces agitation or anxiety

VALIDATING INFORMED CONSENT

The facility must have evidence that sufficient information was provided by the facility so that the resident or resident representative could make an informed decision, voluntarily, free from coercion.

Information that the facility must provide to the resident, or resident representative include but are not limited to:
- What assessed medical needs would be addressed by the use of bed rails;
- The resident's benefits from the use of bed rails and the likelihood of these benefits;
- The resident's risks from the use of bed rails and how these risks will be mitigated; and

- o Alternatives attempted that failed to meet the resident's needs and alternatives considered but not attempted because they were considered to be inappropriate.

*Utilize the Key Elements of Noncompliance found in SOM Appendix PP to evaluate compliance:

§483.25(n)   To cite deficient practice at F700, the surveyor's investigation will generally show that the facility failed to do one or more of the following:

- Identify and use appropriate alternative(s) prior to installing a bed rail;
- Assess the resident for risk of entrapment prior to installing a bed rail;
- Assess the risk versus benefits of using a bed rail and review them with the resident or if applicable, the resident's representative;
- Obtain informed consent for the installation and use of bed rails prior to the installation.
- Ensure appropriate dimensions of the bed, based on the resident's size and weight;
- Ensure correct installation of bed rails, including adherence to manufacturer's recommendations and/or specifications;
- Ensure correct use of an installed bed or side rail; and/or
- Ensure scheduled maintenance of any bed rail in use according to manufacturer's recommendations and specifications.

POST-TRAUMATIC STRESS DISORDER (PTSD) can be a complicated and challenging condition to manage, both for the person suffering the disease and those providing care and treatment. The symptoms of PTSD can lead to a host of psychosocial problems, including job loss, family discord, and substance abuse. Ensuring staff understand and appreciate the many ways stress-related reactions can manifest is essential to establishing a proactive approach to symptom management. Recognizing these reactions as something the affected individual has little ability to control is key to creating a care environment in which healing and quality of life is achievable.

PTSD ASSESSMENT RESOURCES AND TOOLS

- US Department of Veteran's Affairs: National Center for PTSD:
    - https://www.ptsd.va.gov/professional/assessment/screens/index.asp
        - Primary Care PTSD Screen for *DSM-5* (PC-PTSD-5)
        - Trauma Screening Questionnaire (TSQ)
        - American Psychological Association:
    - https://www.apa.org/ptsd-guideline/assessment/index
        - Structured Clinical Interview; PTSD Module (SCID PTSD Module)

ADDITIONAL RESOURCES

Resident Safety/Fall Prevention:

- National Council on Aging National Falls Prevention Resource Center at http://www.ncoa.org/center-for-healthy-aging/falls-resource-center
- Centers for Disease Control and Prevention at http://www.cdc.gov/homeandrecreationalsafety/falls/
- World Health Organization Fall Prevention in Older Age at http://www.who.int/ageing/projects/falls_prevention_older_age/en/
- National Institute of Health- Senior Health at http://nihseniorhealth.gov/falls/aboutfalls/01.html
- Wandering and Elopement Resources National Council of Certified Dementia Practitioners at http://www.nccdp.org

II

Behavioral Health

F740 §483.40 Behavioral health services.

- Each resident must receive and the facility must provide the necessary behavioral health care and services to attain or maintain the highest practicable physical, mental, and psychosocial well-being, in accordance with the comprehensive assessment and plan of care.
- Behavioral health encompasses a resident's whole emotional and mental well-being, which includes, but is not limited to, the prevention and treatment of mental and substance use disorders.

Definitions:

- **"Mental disorder"** is a syndrome characterized by a clinically significant disturbance in an individual's cognition, emotion regulation, or behavior that reflects a dysfunction in the psychological, biological, or developmental processes underlying mental functioning (American Psychiatric Association. Diagnostic and Statistical Manual of Mental Disorders, Fifth edition. Arlington, VA: American Psychiatric Association Publishing, 2013.).

- **"Substance use disorder"** is defined as recurrent use of alcohol and/or drugs that causes clinically and functionally significant impairment, such as health problems or disability.
  (Adapted from: Substance Abuse and Mental Health Services Administration (SAMHSA) definition found at http://www.samhsa.gov/disorders/substance-use).

F741 Behavioral Health

- §483.40(a) The facility must have sufficient staff who provide direct services to residents with the appropriate competencies and skills sets to provide nursing and related services to assure resident safety and attain or maintain the highest practicable physical, mental and psychosocial well-being of each resident, as determined by resident assessments and individual plans of care and considering the number, acuity and diagnoses of the facility's resident population in accordance with §483.70(e).

- These competencies and skills sets include, but are not limited to, knowledge of and appropriate training and supervision for:
    - §483.40(a)(1) Caring for residents with mental and psychosocial disorders, as well as residents with a history of trauma and/or post-traumatic stress disorder, that have been identified in the facility assessment conducted pursuant to
    - §483.40(a)(2) Implementing non-pharmacological interventions.
- **Sufficient Staff to Provide Behavioral Health Care and Services**
    - The facility must address in its **Facility Assessment** under §483.70(e) (F838), the behavioral health needs that can be met and the numbers and types of staff needed to meet these needs.
- §483.40(b) Based on the comprehensive assessment of a resident, the facility must ensure that—
- §483.40(b)(1) A resident who displays or is diagnosed with mental disorder or psychosocial adjustment difficulty, or who has a history of trauma and/or post-traumatic stress disorder, receives appropriate treatment and services to correct the assessed problem or to attain the highest practicable mental and psychosocial well-being;

SKILL AND COMPETENCY OF STAFF

The facility must identify the skills and competencies needed by staff to work effectively with residents (both with and without mental disorders and psychosocial disorders). Staff need to be knowledgeable about implementing non-pharmacological interventions.

- The skills and competencies needed to care for residents should be identified through an evidence-based process that could include the following:
    - An analysis of Minimum Data Set (MDS) data,
    - Review of quality improvement data,
    - Resident-specific and population needs,

- Once identified, staff must be aware of those disease processes that are relevant to enhance psychological and emotional well-being. Competency is established by:
    - Observing the staff's ability to use this knowledge through the demonstration to meet residents' behavioral health care needs; and
    - Staff's ability to communicate and interact with residents in a way that promotes psychosocial and emotional well-being, as well as meaningful engagements.

- Under §483.152 Requirements for approval of a nurse aide training and competency evaluation program, nurse aides are required to complete and provide documentation of training that includes, but is not limited to, competencies in areas such as:
    - Communication and interpersonal skills;
    - Promoting residents' independence;
    - Respecting residents' rights;
    - Caring for the residents' environment;
    - Mental health and social service needs; and
    - Care of cognitively impaired residents.

KEY ELEMENTS OF NONCOMPLIANCE §483.40(a), (a)(1) & (a)(2)

To cite deficient practice at F741, the surveyor's investigation will generally show that the facility failed to:

- Rule out underlying causes for the resident's behavioral health care needs through assessment, diagnosis, and treatment by qualified professionals, such as physicians, including psychiatrists or neurologists;
- Identify competencies and skills sets needed in the facility to work effectively with residents with mental disorders and other behavioral health needs;
- Provide sufficient staff who have the knowledge, training, competencies, and skills sets to address behavioral health care needs;
- Demonstrate reasonable attempts to secure professional behavioral health services, when needed;
- Utilize and implement non-pharmacological approaches to care, based upon the

comprehensive assessment, and in accordance with the resident's abilities, customary daily routine, life-long patterns, interests, preferences, and choices;

- Monitor and provide ongoing assessment of the resident's behavioral health needs, as to whether the interventions are improving or stabilizing the resident's status or causing adverse consequences;
- Attempt alternate approaches to care for the resident's assessed behavioral health needs, if necessary; or
- Accurately document all relevant actions in the resident's medical record.

F742 Behavioral Health
§483.40(b)(1) A resident who displays or is diagnosed with mental disorder or psychosocial adjustment difficulty, or who has a history of trauma and/or post-traumatic stress disorder, receives appropriate treatment and services to correct the assessed problem or to attain the highest practicable mental and psychosocial well-being;

DEFINITIONS §483.40(b) & §483.40(b)(1)
Definitions are provided to clarify terminology related to behavioral health services and the attainment or maintenance of a resident's highest practicable well-being.

"Mental and psychosocial adjustment difficulty" refers to the development of emotional and/or behavioral symptoms in response to an identifiable stressor(s) that has not been the resident's typical response to stressors in the past or an inability to adjust to stressors as evidenced by chronic emotional and/or behavioral symptoms. (Adapted from Diagnostic and Statistical Manual of Mental Disorders - Fifth edition. 2013, American Psychiatric Association.).

INTENT §483.40(b) & §483.40(b)(1)
The intent of this regulation is to ensure that a resident who upon admission, was assessed and displayed or was diagnosed with a mental or psychosocial adjustment difficulty or a history of trauma and/or post-traumatic stress disorder (PTSD), receives the appropriate treatment and services to correct the initial assessed problem or to attain the highest practicable mental and

psychosocial well-being. Residents who were admitted to the nursing home with a mental or psychosocial adjustment difficulty, or who have a history of trauma and/or PTSD, must receive appropriate person-centered and individualized treatment and services to meet their assessed needs.

KEY ELEMENTS OF NONCOMPLIANCE §483.40(b) & §483.40(b)(1)

To cite deficient practice at F742, the surveyor's investigation will generally show that the facility failed to:

- Assess the resident's expressions or indications of distress to determine if services were needed;
- Provide services and individualized care approaches that address the assessed needs of the resident and are within the scope of the resources in the facility assessment;
- Develop an individualized care plan that addresses the assessed emotional and psychosocial needs of the resident;
- Assure that staff consistently implement the care approaches delineated in the care plan;
- Monitor and provide ongoing assessment as to whether the care approaches are meeting the emotional and psychosocial needs of the resident; or
- Review and revise care plans that have not been effective and/or when the resident has a change in condition and accurately document all of these actions in the resident's medical record.

F743 Behavioral Health

§483.40(b)(2) A resident whose assessment did not reveal or who does not have a diagnosis of a mental or psychosocial adjustment difficulty or a documented history of trauma and/or post- traumatic stress disorder does not display a pattern of decreased social interaction and/or increased withdrawn, angry, or depressive behaviors, unless the resident's clinical condition demonstrates that development of such a pattern was unavoidable; and

INTENT §483.40(b)(2)

The intent of this regulation is to ensure that a resident who, upon admission was not assessed or diagnosed with a mental or psychosocial adjustment difficulty or a documented history of trauma and/or post-traumatic stress disorder (PTSD), does not develop patterns of decreased social interaction and/or increased withdrawn, angry, or depressive behaviors while residing in the facility. However, after admission, if the resident is diagnosed with a condition that typically manifests a similar pattern of behaviors, documentation must validate why the pattern was unavoidable (e.g., symptoms did not initially manifest, family was unaware of previous trauma or were unavailable for interview, etc.). Development of an unavoidable pattern of behaviors refers to a situation where the interdisciplinary team, including the resident, their family, and/or resident representative, has completed comprehensive assessments, developed and implemented individualized, person-centered approaches to care through the care-planning process, revised care plans accordingly, and behavioral patterns still manifest.

GUIDANCE §483.40(b)(2)

Nursing home admission can be a stressful experience for a resident, his/her family, and/or representative. Behavioral health is an integral part of a resident's assessment process and care plan development. The assessment and care plan should include goals that are person-centered and individualized to reflect and maximize the resident's dignity, autonomy, privacy, socialization, independence, choice, and safety.

Facility staff must:

- Monitor the resident closely for expressions or indications of distress;
- Assess and plan care for concerns identified in the resident's assessment;
- Accurately document the changes, including the frequency of occurrence and potential triggers in the resident's record;
- Share concerns with the interdisciplinary team (IDT) to determine underlying causes, including differential diagnosis;
- Ensure appropriate follow-up assessment, if needed; and
- Discuss potential modifications to the care plan.

For additional information regarding non-pharmacological interventions, see §483.40(a)(2) (F741), Implementing non-pharmacological interventions.

KEY ELEMENTS OF NONCOMPLIANCE §483.40(b)(2) To cite deficient practice at F743, the surveyor's investigation will generally show the facility failed to:

- Identify that a resident developed decreased social interaction and/or increased withdrawn, angry, or depressive behaviors, and may have made verbalizations indicating these;
- Evaluate whether the resident's distress was attributable to their clinical condition and demonstrate that the change in behavior was unavoidable;
- Ensure an accurate diagnosis of a mental disorder or psychosocial adjustment difficulty, or PTSD was made by a qualified professional;
- Adequately assess and/or develop care plans for services and individualized care approaches that support the needs of residents who develop these patterns;
- Provide services with an individualized care approach that support the needs of residents with these indicators;
- Provide staff with training opportunities related to the person-centered care approaches that have been developed and implemented;
- Assure that staff consistently implement the approaches delineated in the care plan;
- Monitor and provide ongoing assessment as to whether the care approaches are meeting the needs of the resident; or
- Review and revise care planned interventions and accurately document the reason for revision in the resident's medical record.

MENTAL HEALTH RESOURCES
- National Institute of Mental Health:
    - https://www.nimh.nih.gov
- The Mayo Clinic – Mental Health
    - https://www.mayoclinic.org
- The SAMHSA-HRSA Center for Integrated Health Solutions (CIHS):
    - https://www.integration.samhsa.gov

SUBSTANCE USE/ADDICTION RESOURCES
- National Institute on Alcohol Abuse and Alcoholism:
    - https://www.niaaa.nih.gov/
- World Health Organization: Management of Substance Abuse
    - https://www.who.int/substance_abuse/publications/alcohol/en/
- The SAMHSA-HRSA Center for Integrated Health Solutions (CIHS):
    - https://www.integration.samhsa.gov

INTELLECTUAL/DEVELOPMENTAL DISABILITY RESOURCES
- The American Association on Intellectual and Developmental Disabilities (AAIDD):
    - http://www.apdda.org/resources.aspx
    - Administration on Intellectual and Developmental Disabilities (AIDD):
    - www.acl.gov/programs/aidd/index.aspx
    - The Arc of the United States – National/State Chapters for Developmental Disabilities:
    - www.thearc.org

TRAUMATIC BRAIN INJURY (TBI) RESOURCES
- Brain Injury Association of America:
    - https://www.biausa.org/
    - Centers for Disease Control – Traumatic Brain Injury:
    - https://www.cdc.gov/TraumaticBrainInjury/index.html

F744 Behavioral Health

§483.40(b)(3) A resident who displays or is diagnosed with dementia, receives the appropriate treatment and services to attain or maintain his or her highest practicable physical, mental, and psychosocial well-being.

DEFINITIONS §483.40(b)(3)
- Definitions are provided to clarify terminology related to dementia and the attainment or maintenance of a resident's highest practicable well-being.

- **"Dementia"** is a general term to describe a group of symptoms related to loss of memory, judgment, language, complex motor skills, and other intellectual function, caused by the permanent damage or death of the brain's nerve cells, or neurons. However, dementia is not a specific disease. There are many types and causes of dementia with varying symptomology and rates of progression.

    (Adapted from: "About Dementia." Alzheimer's Foundation of America. 30 Nov 2016. Accessed at: https://www.alzfdn.org/AboutDementia/definition.html)

"Highest practicable physical, mental, and psychosocial well-being" is defined as the highest possible level of functioning and well-being, limited by the individual's recognized pathology and normal aging process. Highest practicable is determined through the comprehensive resident assessment and by recognizing and competently and thoroughly addressing the physical, mental or psychosocial needs of the individual.

GUIDANCE §483.40(b)(3)
Providing care for residents living with dementia is an integral part of the person- centered environment, which is necessary to support a high quality of life with meaningful relationships and engagement. Fundamental principles of care for persons living with dementia involve an interdisciplinary approach that focuses holistically on the needs of the resident living with dementia, as well as the needs of the other residents in the nursing home. Additionally, it includes qualified staff that demonstrate the competencies and skills to support residents through the implementation of individualized approaches to care (including direct care and activities) that are directed toward understanding, preventing, relieving, and/or accommodating a resident's distress or loss of abilities.

If there are staffing concerns related to the provision of behavioral health services, refer to §483.40(a) (F741), Sufficient and Competent Staff.
- The facility must provide dementia treatment and services which may include, but are not
- limited to the following:

- Ensuring adequate medical care, diagnosis, and supports based on diagnosis;
- Ensuring that the necessary care and services are person-centered and reflect the resident's goals, while maximizing the resident's dignity, autonomy, privacy, socialization, independence, choice, and safety; and
- Utilizing individualized, non-pharmacological approaches to care (e.g., purposeful and meaningful activities). Meaningful activities are those that address the resident's customary routines, interests, preferences, and choices to enhance the resident's well-being.

KEY ELEMENTS OF NONCOMPLIANCE §483.40(b)(3)
To cite deficient practice at F744, the surveyor's investigation will generally show that the facility failed to:
- Assess resident treatment and service needs through the Resident Assessment Instrument (RAI) process;
- Identify, address, and/or obtain necessary services for the dementia care needs of residents;
- Develop and implement person-centered care plans that include and support the dementia care needs, identified in the comprehensive assessment;
- Develop individualized interventions related to the resident's symptomology and rate of progression (e.g., providing verbal, behavioral, or environmental prompts to assist a resident with dementia in the completion of specific tasks);
- Review and revise care plans that have not been effective and/or when the resident has a change in condition;
- Modify the environment to accommodate resident care needs; or
- Achieve expected improvements or maintain the expected stable rate of decline.

DEMENTIA ASSESSMENT RESOURCES AND TOOLS
- **Alzheimer's Association:** www.alz.org
- **Pioneer Network:** www.pioneernetwork.org

Tools: Sometimes used in addition to the MDS 3.0, Section C - Cognition
- **Global Deterioration Scale**
- **Dementia Screening Indicator (Barnes, et al.)**
- **Geriatric Depression Scale**

STAFF EDUCATION, TRAINING, AND CERTIFICATION

1. **Certified Dementia Practitioner**
   - https://www.nccdp.org/cdp.htm
2. **Alzheimer's Association - EssentiALZ Certification Program**
   - https://www.alz.org/professionals/professional-providers/certification-program
3. Dementia Care Specialist Certification
   - https://www.crisisprevention.com/What-We-Do/Dementia-Care-Specialists/Dementia-Care-Specialist-Certification
4. **Oasis** – Dr. Susan Wehry's Curriculum for Dementia Certification
   - http://www.oasis.today/online-training.html

PRE-ADMISSIONS SCREENING AND RESIDENT REVIEW (PASARR)

F645 COORDINATION

- **Incorporating the recommendations from the PASARR level II determination and the PASARR evaluation report into a resident's assessment, care planning, and transitions of care.**
- **Referring all level II residents and all residents with newly evident or possible serious mental disorder, intellectual disability, or a related condition for level II resident review upon a <u>significant change</u> in status assessment.**

F646

PASARR - Significant Change

- **§483.20(k)(4) A nursing facility must notify the state mental health authority or state intellectual disability authority, as applicable, promptly after a significant change in the <u>mental or physical</u> condition of a resident who has mental illness or intellectual disability for resident review.**
- **"Significant Change" is a major decline or improvement in a resident's status that:**
  - **1) will not normally resolve itself without intervention by staff or by implementing standard disease-related clinical interventions; the decline is not considered "self-limiting"**

- (NOTE: Self-limiting is when the condition will normally resolve itself without further intervention or by staff implementing standard clinical interventions to resolve the condition.);
- 2) impacts more than one area of the resident's health status; and
- 3) requires interdisciplinary review and/or revision of the care plan.

*This does not change the facility's requirement to immediately consult with a resident's physician of changes as required under 42 CFR §483.10(i)(14), F580.

TIMEFRAMES FOR PASARR COMPLIANCE:

The timeframes are:
- The Level I PASARR SCREEN must be completed prior to admission to a RHCF for every person, for any reason and any length of stay.
- As soon as a person has been **newly diagnosed** with a mental illness and/or intellectual disability/developmental disability.

PASARR Technical Assistance Center: The PASRR Technical Assistance Center helps states fulfill the goals of Preadmission Screening and Resident Review. Consult their website for information and assistance in complying with the Federal PASAAR requirements.

https://www.pasrrassist.org/

III

FACILITY ASSESSMENT

Assessing Needed Care and Services and Staff Competency

F838

FACILITY ASSESSMENT

- **The facility must conduct and document a facility-wide assessment to determine what resources are necessary to care for its residents competently during both day-to-day operations and emergencies.**
  - **Review and update at least annually, whenever there is, or the facility plans for, any change that would require a substantial modification to any part of this assessment;**
  - **Must address or include a facility-based and community-based risk assessment, utilizing an all-hazards approach;**
  - **The results of the facility assessment must be used, in part, to establish and update the IPCP, its policies and/or protocols to include a system for preventing, identifying, reporting, investigating, and controlling infections and communicable diseases for residents, staff, and visitors.**
  - **Note: a community-based risk assessment should include review for risk of infections (e.g., Multidrug-resistant organisms- MDROS) and communicable diseases such as tuberculosis and influenza. Appropriate resident tuberculosis screening should be performed based on state requirements.**

F741 GUIDANCE §483.40(a), (a)(1) & (a)(2) Sufficient Staff to Provide Behavioral Health Care and Services The facility must address in its **Facility Assessment** under §483.70(e) (F838), the behavioral health needs that can be met and the numbers and types of staff needed to meet these needs.

F725 §483.35 Nursing Services

As required under Administration at F838, §483.70(e) an assessment of the resident population is the foundation of the facility assessment and determination of the level of sufficient staff needed. It must include an evaluation of diseases, conditions, physical, functional or cognitive limitations of the resident population's, acuity (the level of severity of residents' illnesses, physical, mental and cognitive limitations and conditions) and any other pertinent information about the residents that may affect the services the facility must provide. The assessment of the resident population should drive staffing decisions and inform the facility about what skills and competencies staff must possess in order to deliver the necessary care required by the residents being served.

EVALUATING MEDICATION MANAGEMENT/UNNECESSARY DRUGS

To determine if each resident receives:
- Only those medications that are clinically indicated in the dose and for the duration to meet his or her assessed needs;
- Non-pharmacological approaches when clinically indicated, in an effort to reduce the need for or the dose of a medication; and
- Gradual dose reduction attempts for antipsychotics (unless clinically contraindicated) and tapering of other medications, when clinically indicated, in an effort to discontinue the use or reduce the dose of the medication.

Clinical Documentation

Did staff describe the behavior in the medical record with enough specific detail of the actual situation to permit underlying cause identification to the extent possible?
- Onset
- Duration
- Intensity
- Possible precipitating events
- Environmental triggers
- Related factors (appearance, alertness, etc.)

Clinical Care and Service Assessment
- Staff and Resident/Family Education and Support Services
- Identification/Recruitment of Medical (MD/NP/RNs) Professionals Proficient in Mental Health/Addictions
- Liaisons with Psychiatric/Psychological Service Providers
- Service Agreements with Community Mental Health Service and Support Organizations (i.e., AA, NA, etc.)
- Revision and Enhancement of Therapeutic Activity to Include Self-Help, Self-Awareness, Peer Support, and Educational/Vocational Opportunities.

Attachment A
Rules of Participation Requirements by Phase

Phase 1 - November 28, 2016

1. §483.1 Basis and scope
2. §483.5 Definitions
3. §483.10 Resident rights
4. §483.12 Freedom from abuse, neglect, and exploitation
5. §483.15 Admission, transfer, and discharge rights
6. §483.20 Resident assessment
7. §483.21 Comprehensive person-centered care planning
8. §483.24 Quality of life
9. §483.25 Quality of care
10. §483.30 Physician services
11. §483.35 Nursing services
12. §483.40 Behavioral health services
    1. (d) Comprehensive assessment and medically related social services
13. §483.45 Pharmacy services
14. §483.50 Laboratory, radiology, and other diagnostic services
15. §483.55 Dental services
16. §483.60 Food and nutrition services
17. §483.65 Specialized rehabilitative services
18. §483.70 Administration
19. §483.75 Quality assurance and performance improvement
    1. (h) Disclosure of information
    2. (I) Sanctions
20. §483.80 Infection control
21. §483.90 Physical environment
22. §483.95 Training requirements
    1. (c) Abuse, neglect, and exploitation training

2. (g)(1) Regarding in-service training,
3. (g)(2) dementia management & abuse prevention training,
4. (g)(4) care of the cognitively impaired
5. (h) Training of feeding assistants

Phase 2 - November 28, 2017

1. 483.10 Resident rights
    1. (g)(4)(ii) – (v) Providing contact information for State and local advocacy organizations, Medicare and Medicaid eligibility information, Aging and Disability Resources Center and Medicaid Fraud Control Unit
2. 483.12 Freedom from abuse, neglect, and exploitation
    1. (b)(5) Reporting crimes/1150B
3. 483.15 Admission, transfer, and discharge rights
    1. (c)(2) Transfer/Discharge Documentation
4. 483.21 Comprehensive person-centered care planning
    1. (a) Baseline care plan
5. 483.35 Nursing services
    1. Specific usage of the Facility Assessment at §483.70(e) in the determination of sufficient number and competencies for staff
6. 483.40 Behavioral health services
7. 483.45 Pharmacy services
    1. (c)(2) Medical chart review
    2. (e) Psychotropic drugs
8. 483.55 Dental services
    1. (a)(3) and (a)(5) Loss or damage of dentures and policy for referral (b)(3) and
    2. (b)(4) Referral for dental services regarding loss or damaged dentures
9. 483.60 Food and nutrition services
    1. (a) As linked to Facility Assessment at §483.70(e)
    2. (a)(2)(I) Dietitians designated to after the effective date— Built in implementation date of 1 year following the effective date of the final rule.
10. 483.70 Administration

1. (e) Facility assessment
11. 483.75 Quality assurance and performance improvement
    1. (a)(2) Initial QAPI Plan must be provided to State Agency Surveyor at annual survey
12. 483.80 Infection control
    1. (a) As linked to Facility Assessment at §483.70(e)
    2. (a)(3) Antibiotic stewardship
13. 483.90 Physical environment
    1. (h)(5) Policies regarding smoking

Phase 3 - November 28, 2019

1. 483.12 Freedom from abuse, neglect, and exploitation
   1. (b)(4) Coordination with QAPI Plan
2. 483.21 Comprehensive person-centered care planning
   1. (b)(3)(iii) Trauma informed care
3. 483.25 Quality of care
   1. (m) Trauma informed care
4. 483.40 Behavioral health services
   1. (a)(1) As related to residents with a history of trauma Deadline and/or post-traumatic stress disorder
5. 483.60 Food and nutrition services
   1. (a)(1)(iv) Dietitians hired or contracted with prior to effective date—Built in implementation date of 5 years following effective date of the final rule.
   2. (a)(2)(I) Director of food & nutrition services designated to serve prior to effective—Built in implementation date Deadline of 5 years following the effective date of the final rule.
6. 483.70 Administration
   1. (d)(3) Governing body responsibility of QAPI program
7. 483.75 Quality assurance and performance improvement
   1. (g)(1) QAA committee the addition of the ICPO
8. 483.80 Infection control

1. (b) Infection "preventionist" (IP)
2. (c) IP participation on QAA committee
9. 483.85 Compliance and Ethics program
10. 483.90 Physical environment
    1. (f)(1) Call system from each resident's bedside
11. 483.95 Training requirements

REFERENCES

State Operations Manual Appendix PP - Guidance to Surveyors for Long Term Care Facilities (Rev. 11-22-17)
https://www.cdc.gov/nchs/data/hus/2017/092.pdg
https://assets.aarp.org/rgcenter/il/fs10r_homes.pdf
https://www.nytimes.com/2017/10/24/science/medicaid-cutbacks-elderly-nursing-homes.html
https://www.cms.gov/medicare/provider-enrollment-and-certifcation/guidanceforlawsandregulations/nursing-homes.html

ABOUT THE AUTHOR

Barbara Speedling

*Personally dedicated to the creation of meaningful,
satisfying lives for all those who rely on another's care*

An inspirational and motivational speaker, Barbara is an author, educator and management consultant at the forefront of person-centered care.

An innovator with more than 30 years of practical experience within the adult care community, she is the expert providers turn to when they want to ensure that the services they provide meet not only the physical needs of their residents, but their emotional and psychosocial needs as well. Working from a core belief in the dignity and individuality of all people, Barbara has helped countless adult care communities implement her unique training and education programs that:

- ✓ Improve the quality of care for those living with Alzheimer's disease
- ✓ Bring better quality of life to such residents, as well as to those who live with disease-related dementia, a mental illness, or a brain injury
- ✓ Encourage staffers to use newly developed cultural empathy to form better relationships with those in their care
- ✓ Offer new strategies for promoting harmony among increasingly diverse, younger and assertive populations
- ✓ Open new pathways to maintaining regulatory compliance
- ✓ Support leadership and organizational development

In addition to her degree in healthcare administration, Barbara is an accomplished musician and artist. She uses those talents to develop new and creative ways of reaching out to those who are cognitively diminished. She was also certified in 2015 by Dr. Susan Wehry as a Master Trainer for the OASIS education program for improved care of residents with dementia.

The author of two books devoted to common sense advice for meeting the holistic needs of an increasingly diverse and challenging community, both *Why is Grandma Screaming* and *Toward Better Behavior: Yours Mine & Everyone Else's* are now widely distributed to staff members at community, residential and long-term care facilities across the country and in Canada.

_____

www.ingramcontent.com/pod-product-compliance
Lightning Source LLC
Chambersburg PA
CBHW081649220526
45468CB00009B/2594